Kawasaki Disease: A Slowly Developed Health Issue

David L. Jonathan

Table of Contents

Introduction

Parents should always closely observe their children's characteristics - both mental and physical. Sometimes children suffer from prolonged fever or develop unusual physical changes, like swollen blood vessels or strawberry tongue. In this case, you should rush to the doctors without making any delay because your children might be suffering from Kawasaki disease.

The condition can develop heart problems in children and can also cause inflammation of blood vessels (vasculitis). Since blood vessels include veins, arteries, and capillaries, hence inflammation can also disrupt the supply of oxygenated blood to the heart by blocking coronary arteries. As a result, the patient may be affected by severe heart complications, such as bulging and weakening of the artery wall (an aneurysm), heart muscle inflammation (myocarditis) and abnormal heart rhythm (dysrhythmia).

As the name suggests, this rare but serious disease was first diagnosed in Japan in 1967 and was named after the Japanese pediatrician Tomisaku Kawasaki. The matter of concern is that nowadays Kawasaki disease, also known as "mucocutaneous lymph node syndrome", is found all over the world especially in boys. Therefore, don't ignore and keep your children safe.

Chapter 1- Background of Kawasaki Disease

Kawasaki disease (KD) is a serious disorder of an acute febrile vasculitis syndrome with an onset in early childhood. Another name by which it is sometimes called is "periarteritis nodosa". As history states, in 1967 around 50 cases of children been had been reported to be diagnosed with a unique disease at the Tokyo Red Cross Medical Center in Japan. Dr. Tomisaku Kawasaki was the first to describe this unusual epidemic and hence this disease was named after him. These young patients were admitted with the complaint of rash, inflammation of lips and oral cavity, fever, edema of feet and hands, cervical lymphadenitis, erythema, and conjunctival infection. Initially, the condition was assumed to be self-limited and benign. However, test reports revealed that about 2% of patients died later on who were suffering from this disease. Most of the death occurred among children below the age of 2 years. They died either during their recovery stage or when they had become healthy again. According to the post-mortem reports, the cause of the sudden death was a myocardial infarction (MI) with total thrombotic occlusion of coronary artery aneurysms (CAAs).

In the United States, Melish et al were the first to report about Kawasaki disease in 1976. The report was based on examining 12 children from Honolulu in the years 1971 - 1973. Although the outbreak of this condition was seen in Japan but it is now found all over the world. In the United States, Kawasaki disease has successfully outshined acute rheumatic fever as the primary cause of acquired heart disease among children of less than 5 years old. On the other hand, in the developing countries, this disease is seen to be the main cause of acquired heart problems among children and is also a potential risk factor for ischemic heart disease in the adult.

As shown by the echocardiographic studies, approximately 20 - 25% of children who remain untreated tend to develop sequelae starting from aneurysm formation or asymptomatic coronary artery ectasia to very large CAAs with MI, thrombosis, and sudden death. The mortality rate in this type of cases is 0.1 - 2%. The risk of developing cardiac problems can be reduced to 5% by administrating intravenous immunoglobulin (IVIG) at an early stage. Although the biliary tract, kidneys, and pancreas have been infected with inflammatory infiltration, yet significant sequelae does not persist in the tissues of these organs.

The diagnosis of Kawasaki disease is utterly based on the group of clinical findings since there is no pathognomonic clinical outcome and also there is no specific test available for diagnosing Kawasaki disease. The most common clinical feature of this illness is prolonged fever accompanied by other 4 or 5 major characteristics.

In some special cases or incomplete cases, laboratory examinations support the diagnosis. This because feverish patients in these cases seemed to be suffering from Kawasaki disease but do not fulfill the criteria of diagnosis and also do not have other unknown reason of their illness.

Whenever patients experience the symptoms of Kawasaki disease, they should never delay the diagnosis. Otherwise, this may lead to coronary lesions and other serious complications although many patients can recover without facing any kind of physical activity inadequacy. Patients must be mentally prepared for all types of typical and unusual testing of the disease in order to get the maximum output from the diagnosis. The ideal time to start the therapy is within 7 – 10 days from the onset of fever.

It is evident that around 25% of KD patients who are left untreated can develop coronary artery aneurysms which can remain clinically dormant for many years. During this time, thrombose inducing myocardial infarction can also occur. Recently, children of Western Europe, United States, and Asia are suffering from heart diseases for which the most common etiology is Kawasaki disease. Therefore, whenever a cardiologist deals with a case of coronary artery aneurysms in young adults, he/she should also consider the possibility of untreated KD in the patient's children for which the heart disease may have occurred.

Aspirin and IVIG have been proven to be the most effective therapies to treat KD. However, there are many questions regarding the effectiveness of aspirin. Patients with disease refractory to IVIG are prescribed by the doctors to use infliximab, corticosteroids, and other such agents.

Chapter 2- Get Your Facts Straight

Statistics of KD

According to the estimation of the Kawasaki Disease Foundation (KDF), each year in the United States approximately 4,200 children suffer from Kawasaki disease. In 1999, American Family Physician published a review claiming that Kawasaki disease is the main reason behind the acquired heart disease among the children of some developed countries, such as the United States.

Kawasaki disease can become an alarming issue if left untreated. However, if treated early, they tend to recover very soon, almost within few weeks, without facing any serious heart complications. Patients experience relapses very rarely, although neglecting the condition can eventually lead to issues with the arteries of the heart and cause death from heart attack.

Classification of KD

Vasculitis, or inflammation, of the veins and arteries, takes place throughout the body. Generally, this results from the enhanced generation of the cells of the immune system to an **autoimmunity** or **pathogen**. The classification of the systemic vasculitides is done based on the type of cells related to proliferation and also on the damage of special types of tissue occurring within the arterial walls and veins.

Kawasaki disease is believed to be a **necrotizing** vasculitis under the scheme of the classification system. This is also known as "necrotizing angiitis" and this may be historically identified by the presence of fibrosis, necrosis (tissue death) and proliferation of cells related to the inflammations formed on the inner side of the vascular wall. **Henoch-Schönlein purpura, polyarteritis nodosa, Churg-Strauss syndrome** and **granulomatosis with polyangiitis** are some of the diseases that introduce necrotizing vasculitis.

The harmful Kawasaki disease can further be categorized as a medium-sized vessel vasculitis. This vasculitis can affect medium- and small-sized blood vessels, for instance, the tiny cutaneous vasculature, that is the arteries and veins in the skin. This vasculature is so tiny that its diameter only ranges from 50 to 100 μm.

Kawasaki disease mostly attacks the children below the age of 18. For this reason, this condition is considered to be the main childhood disorder that is associated with vasculitis. Recently, an evaluation of vasculitides based on the consensus of this condition happening to children evolves the categorization method for these disorders. This is done to differentiate them and recommend a better and appropriate set of diagnostic standards for each. Kawasaki disease is again considered to be the principal medium-sized vessel vasculitis within this categorization of childhood vasculitides.

The disease is also considered to be an autoimmune form of vasculitis, but this is not related to ANCA antibodies. Unlike KD, other vasculitic disorders are related to the ANCA antibodies, for instance, Churg-Strauss syndrome, granulomatosis with polyangiitis and microscopic polyangiitis. In order to treat the condition appropriately, this classification is very significant.

Risk Factors of KD

Anything that can increase the risk of enhancing a condition or a disease is considered to be a risk factor. For instance, we all know that people who smoke regularly are more prone to develop different kinds of cancers. Hence, regular smoking is known to be a risk factor for developing cancer. Likewise, there are three things that are considered to make your child more prone to Kawasaki disease, these are:

i. **Ethnic background** – Children who have Asian ancestry, such as Chinese, Korean or Japanese, are more prone to be suffering from Kawasaki disease compared to people of other belts.

ii. **Age** – Children of ages between 2 to 5 years are mostly likely to develop Kawasaki disease than people of other age groups.

iii. **Gender** – Anyone can develop Kawasaki disease. But compared to girls, boys are more prone to be infected with this disease.

Chapter 3- Observe and Act Accordingly

Signs and Symptoms

The most common symptom of Kawasaki disease is a very high fever which is so stubborn that it does not go away with usual treatment, such as taking ibuprofen or paracetamol (acetaminophen). It is the most prominent sign of having Kawasaki disease and is a characteristic symbol of the acute phase of the disease. The fever is usually remittent, higher than 39 – 40°C and also makes the patient extremely irritability. In recent cases, it has been reported that patients with unusual or incomplete Kawasaki disease suffer from this condition. However, it is not evident in all of the cases. The first day the patient gets a fever is said to be the first day of illness. In average the duration of fever is usually 1 to 2 weeks. If the patient is left untreated, the fever may be prolonged to 3 to 4 weeks or even more. Long lasting fever is believed to be linked to the higher occurrence of cardiac complications. It does not stop with the consumption of antibiotics but partially responds to antipyretic drugs. However, with the introduction of proper treatment, such as aspirin and intravenous immunoglobulin, the patient can get rid of fever within 2 days.

After fever the most common symptom reported to be was bilateral **conjunctival inflammation**. It is not painful and does not accompany suppuration but it often involves the bulbar conjunctivae. The symptom usually starts soon after the beginning of fever when the disease at its acute stage. If the slit-lamp examination is carried out, then the presence of **anterior uveitis** can be found. Also, the occurrence of **iritis** is not very surprising. Another example of eye manifestation is the **erratic precipitation.** These are visible by a slit-lamp examination but most of the time these are very tiny to be visible to the naked eye.

Signs and symptoms of Kawasaki disease often include a set of oral manifestations. Most of the time, the characteristic physical transformations are swollen lips (**edema**) along with bleeding and fissures (vertical cracking). In addition, the mucosa of the oropharynx may turn bright red and the tongue may become like a "strawberry tongue" with the appearance of marked erythema and protruding gustative papillae. These oral manifestations occur because of **fibrinoid necrosis** and **necrotizing micro vasculitis.** Around 50% to 75% of patients are infected with **cervical lymphadenopathy.** On the other hand, the rest of the features occur in an average of 90% of the patients. However, sometimes the symptoms can be present dominantly.

The definition of the diagnostic criteria explains that minimum of one impaired lymph node must be greater than or equal to 1.5 cm in diameter must be present. Lymph nodes which are affected are not- fluctuant, cause you less pain and are nonsuppurative. You can also notice erythema of the adjacent skin. Children with neck adenitis and fever who are resistant to antibiotics must do the tests of Kawasaki disease assuming as an important procedure of differential diagnoses. Changes can be seen in the peripheral extremities, such as erythema soles and palms, during the acute phase of the Kawasaki disease. Often this is conveyed by beefy, brawny, painful edema of the dorsum of the feet and hands and this also strikes with sharp confinement. For this reason, child patients do not want to hold things in their hands or carry weight in their feet. Later on, when the patients are in the sub-acute phase or are recovering, desquamation of the toes and fingers often starts in the periungual region. This happens within 2 to 3 weeks after the commencement of the fever and even sometimes extends to include the soles and the palms. Approximately 11% of children who are suffering from the disease may have their skins continue to peel for many years. Soon after 1 to 2 months from the starting of the fever, development of deep crosswise grooves across the nails can be seen, also called **Beau's lines**, and the nails shed off rarely.

The diffuse macular popular erythematous rash is the most usual cutaneous manifestation. This is very nonspecific. The rash changes over time and has a characteristic tendency to be located in the trunk. This may further spread in areas, such as perineum, face, and extremities. Reports of various other forms of cutaneous lesions have been known. These may include purpuric lesions, papular, scarlatiniform, multiform-like erythema, and utriculiform. In addition, micro pustules have been known to be reported. This can be usually observed until the fifth day of the fever and can be polymorphic. But it can never be vesicular or bullous. In many organs during the acute stage of Kawasaki disease, systemic inflammatory changes can be seen. Arthritis, swelling, joint pain (**arthralgia**) can also be formed in the body. Lymphadenitis, valvulitis, aseptic meningitis, hepatitis, pericarditis, myocarditis, pneumonitis, and diarrhea can be present and these are also manifested by the existence of inflammatory cells in the cells which are affected. If these conditions are not treated, then eventually some of the symptoms will concede. However, coronary artery aneurysms will not recover. This will result in disability because of myocardial infarction or in a prominent risk of death. If you treat the disease at an early stage, this risk can be avoided to a great length and you will recover soon.

Other cases of reported nonspecific symptoms include seizure, sputum, cough, vomiting, rhinorrhea and headache. The complete progression of the disease can be grouped into 3 clinical phases:

i) **Acute febrile phase** – This phase normally stays for 1 to 2 weeks. The characteristic symptoms of this stage include fever, erythema, and swelling of feet and hands, conjunctiva injection, diarrhea, rash, hepatic dysfunction, aseptic meningitis, cervical adenopathy and erythema of the oral mucosa. Pericardial effusion can be found at this time but myocarditis is commonly seen at this stage. Echocardiography cannot generally detect aneurysms, although coronary arteritis may be present.

ii) **Subacute phase** – The onset of this stage causes rash, fever and lymphadenopathy to resolve at around 1 to 2 weeks after the beginning of fever. However, anorexia, conjunctival infection and irritability still persist. At this stage, thrombocytosis and the peeling of the skin of toes and fingers are usually seen. This generally persists for around 4 weeks after the beginning of fever. This stage is very lethal as during this time patients normally develop coronary artery aneurysms. Therefore, the risk of sudden death of patients is the highest.

iii) **Convalescent stage** – This stage starts at the disappearance of all the clinical signs and symptoms of sickness from the disease. The stage continues until the rate of sedimentation goes back to normal level. Generally, convalescent stage lasts 6 to 8 weeks after the starting of the ailment.

The signs and symptoms of each stage and other clinical presentations of the disorder differ from adults to that of children. This is because the lymph nodes in adults are more affected than the children. About 65% of adults get affected by hepatitis while only 10% of children suffer from this complication. When only 24% to 38% of children get affected by arthralgia, on the other hand, 61% of adults suffer from this condition. Classical signs and symptoms may be absent in few of the patients. They may produce an atypical presentation of the illness. This usually happens to young infants particularly and, hence, these patients are especially are more prone to develop cardiac artery aneurysms.

Complications

Kawasaki disease can lead to serious complications in children if left untreated. One of the complications that may result involves cardiac problems. Other complications may also stir up and may result in serious consequences. Nevertheless, if the children are treated effectively then only a few patients may experience lasting damage.

- **Cardiac** - The most important issue of Kawasaki disease which is worth discussing is the cardiac complications. It is the primary reason behind the heart diseases acquired in childhood, especially in Japan and the United States. In around 20% to 25% of untreated child patients, coronary heart aneurysms take place as a sequel of the vasculitis. Most of the time, coronary artery dilation or aneurysms take place within 4 weeks of starting of the illness and the problem is detected for the first time at an average of 10 days of the onset. Aneurysms are categorized into giant (diameter is greater than 8 mm), medium (the diameter ranges from 5 to 8 mm) and small (the internal diameter of the wall of the vessel is less than 5mm). Between 18 and 25 days after the starting of the illness, fusiform aneurysms and saccular are normally developed.

Even when a high dose of IVIG regimens is administered within the first 10 days of the disease, 1% of the children affected with Kawasaki disease get giant aneurysms and 5% of children get at least dilation of the transient coronary artery. Death can happen due to rupture of a large coronary artery aneurysm or because of myocardial infarction subordinate to the formation of blood clot. After the onset of the disease, death commonly occurs within 2 to 12 weeks. A scientist could identify several risk factors that can cause coronary artery aneurysms. This includes low hemoglobin concentrations, persistent fever even after IVIG therapy, a high count of white blood cell, low concentration of albumin, high CRP concentrations, male sex, age below 1 year and a high count of the band. Kawasaki disease can result in coronary artery lesions that can dynamically change with time. The resolution has been observed 1 to 2 years after the starting of the illness in half of the vessels in case of coronary aneurysms. The recovery process of the vessel wall results in the narrowing of the coronary artery. This often leads to noteworthy obstruction of the blood vessels. Also, because of this, the heart cannot receive enough blood and oxygen. Eventually, this can lead to the death of the tissue of the heart muscle (myocardial infarction).

The main cause of death from the Kawasaki disease is MI which is instigated by thrombotic occlusion in a stenotic, aneurysmal or both stenotic and aneurysmal coronary artery. During the first year just after the starting of the disease, patients have the highest risk of developing MI. Different symptoms can be seen in adults with MI than in children with MI. The primary and the most common symptoms in older children include chest pain, unrest vomiting, shock and abdominal pain. Many of these children experience the attack taking place while they are asleep or are at rest. Around one-third of the attacks in children were seen to be asymptomatic. Valvular insufficiencies, especially of tricuspid valves and mitral, are often seen during the acute phase of Kawasaki disease. This happens due to inflammation of the heart muscle or inflammation of the heart valve-induced myocardial dysfunction, even without the involvement of coronary issues. Most of the time, these lesions go away with the resolution of the acute illness, although a very small collection of lesions persist and progress. In addition, there is late-start mitral or aortic insufficiency which is caused by the deformation or thickening of fibrosis valves. This happens during the time ranging from several months to even years after the beginning of the Kawasaki disease. Valve replacement may be recommended for some of the lesions.

- **Other** – Other complications of Kawasaki disease have been talked about, for instance, aneurysm of other arteries: axillary artery aneurysm, aortic aneurysm, brachiocephalic artery aneurysm, with a higher number of reported cases involving the abdominal aorta, renal artery aneurysm, and aneurysm of femoral and iliac arteries. Further vascular complications include increased thickness of the wall and reduced distensibility of carotid arteries, brachioradialis artery, and the aorta. Eventually, change in vascular tone secondary to endothelial dysfunction can be seen. Moreover, child patients with the Kawasaki disease may have more dangerous cardiovascular risk profile, like obesity, high blood pressure, and an abnormal serum lipid profile. This kind of patients may or may not experience coronary artery complications.

Complications observed in Henoch-Schönlein purpura, such as the acute abdomen, colon swelling, intestinal obstruction, intestinal pseudo-obstruction and intestinal ischemia, are similar to the gastrointestinal complications of the Kawasaki disease.

Since the 1980s, changes in the eye associated with the disorder have been described to be found as optic neuritis, uveitis, conjunctival hemorrhage, iridocyclitis, amaurosis, and ocular artery obstruction. This can also be observed as necrotizing vasculitis that is developing into peripheral gangrene.

The neurological complications in lesions of per central nervous system have often been recorded. The neurological complications include cerebral hypoperfusion, meningoencephalitis, subdural effusion, cerebral ischemia and cerebellar infarction, infarct manifesting with seizures, chorea, lethargy and coma, hemiplegia, mental confusion, or even a cerebral infarction with no neurological manifestations. Further neurological complications from the involvement of the cranial nerve are known to be facial palsy, sensorineural and ataxia. The behavioral changes that are assumed to be caused by localized cerebral hypoperfusion can accompany with learning deficits, attention deficit, emotional disorders (night terrors, emotional lability, and fear of night) and internalization issues which include aggressive behavior, depression and anxious.

Chapter 4- Why It Happens & What to Do?

Causes of KD

It is still unknown what exactly cause the Kawasaki disease. The disorder is more accurately known as "Kawasaki syndrome". This has a similarity with all the autoimmune diseases, that is, it is presumably caused by the interaction between genetic and environmental factors, most probably during an infection. No one really knows the specific cause, but primarily current theory suggests immunological factors to be the main causes. Although there is a debate on whether the cause is a superantigen or a conventional antigenic substance, but evidence increasingly hold infectious etiology to be responsible for this disease. According to the reports given by the researchers of Boston Children's Hospital, it has been found in some studies that the occurrence of the Kawasaki disease is associated with the recent exposure to carpet washing or house near an area of stagnant water. However, this hypothesis of cause and effect has not been established yet.

Other analytical data indicate that Kawasaki disease is clearly associated with tropospheric wind patterns. It has been seen that the wind blowing from the central Asia is correlated with Kawasaki disease that affects the children of San Diego, Japan, and Hawaii. The relation with tropospheric winds has been shown to be curbed at seasonal and inter-annual timescales by the El Niño - Southern Oscillation phenomenon, which further indicates water-borne pathogen is the agent responsible for the Kawasaki disease. Scientists are putting their best effort to find out the suspected pathogen in air filters that can fly at an altitude over Japan.

A correlation has been found between the cause of the disease and an SNP in the ITPKC gene. This gene codes an enzyme that regulates the activation of the T-cell negatively. Regardless of where the child patients are living, Japanese children are always more prone to the disease that other children. This suggests that genetic susceptibility is somehow is behind all these. After an investigation, the HLA-B51 serotype has been found to be related to endemic occurrences of the disease.

Diagnosis of KD

There is no existence of any laboratory tests for Kawasaki disease. This can only be diagnosed by observing medical signs and symptoms (clinically). It is not very easy to launch the diagnosis, especially in the early stage of the condition. Often children are not sent for diagnosis until they have visited many health-care providers. Several other serious diseases, such as childhood mercury poisoning (infantile acrodynia), juvenile idiopathic arthritis, toxic shock syndrome and scarlet fever, can cause similar signs and symptoms and, hence, must be considered during the differential diagnosis. Generally, in order to establish the diagnosis five days of fever along with 4 out of 5 of the following diagnostic criteria must be met. The criteria are:

1. a rash on the trunk
2. red eyes (conjunctiva infection)
3. erythema of the oral cavity or the lips or cracking of the lips skin
4. erythema or swelling of the feet or hands
5. at least 15 mm of the swollen lymph node in the neck

According to the Kuo mnemonic, there is a rapid memory method to remember diagnosis criteria: "1 dry mouth, 2 red eyes, 3 fingers touch neck lymph node swelling, 4 limbs change, and 5 much skin rash with fever more than 5 days".

Many children, particularly children, do not exhibit the above diagnostic criteria even though they suffer from Kawasaki disease eventually. In fact, many doctors and experts recommend treating for Kawasaki disease even if the patient suffers from only 3 days of fever and only 3 diagnostic criteria have met. They do this especially when other tests show abnormalities similar to that of with Kawasaki disease. Furthermore, the diagnosis can be carried out completely by the detection of coronary artery aneurysms in the appropriate clinical instrumental settings.

Some Required Investigations

A list of investigations is required to identify the causes responsible for Kawasaki disease. A thorough physical examination will reveal many of the criteria enlisted above.

1. *Blood tests*

- **A complete blood count** will help identity normocytic anemia   which may eventually become thrombocytosis.
- The **rate of erythrocyte sedimentation** will be increased.
- Increased level of **C-reactive protein** will be seen.
- **Tests of liver function** may reveal a trace of hepatic inflammation and low levels of serum albumin.

2. *Other tests (optional)*

- **Electrocardiogram** may help you show a trace of ventricular dysfunction, or sometimes even show arrhythmia due to myocarditis.

- **An echocardiogram** will reveal elusive coronary artery changes, any aneurysms at a later date.

- **Biopsy** of the temporal artery

- **Lumbar puncture** may reveal traces of aseptic meningitis.

- **Urinalysis** will help you find out protein and white blood cells in the urine (proteinuria and pyuria) without the trace of any bacterial growth.

- Historically **angiography** was used to detect coronary artery aneurysms and stayed the gold standard for their detection. However, today it is rarely used unless echocardiography has already detected coronary artery aneurysms.

- **Computerized tomography** or **ultrasound** can be used to identify enlargement (hydrops) of the gall bladder.

Treatment of KD

Children suffering from Kawasaki disease must be admitted to the hospital and should be treated properly by a doctor or a physician who has experience dealing with this disease. When admitted in any academic medical center, the treatment is divided among pediatric rheumatology, pediatric cardiology, and pediatric infectious disease specialists. However, there has not been any report about a specific infectious agent yet. It is advised to start the treatment as soon as the illness is being diagnosed. This is to avoid damage to the coronary arteries. The standard treatment for Kawasaki disease is Intravenous immunoglobulin (IVIG) which is administered in patients at high doses to achieve marked improvement within a very short time (preferably within 24 hours). Even after this of the patient still has a fever, then doctors may consider giving an additional dose to the patient. It is very rare that a third dose is being administered to the child. In terms of preventing coronary artery aneurysms, IVIG is the most useful and effective option by itself when given within the first 7 days of the starting of the fever.

Alternately, salicylate therapy (especially aspirin) can be considered as an important component of the treatment, although it is questioned by many. If salicylates are used alone then no significant effect is seen as IVIG. The therapy of aspirin begins with high doses until the fever recedes. After that, it is continued at a low dose when the patient is discharged and sent home. This usually continues for 2 months to prevent the formation of blood clots. Generally, aspirin is not recommended for children due to its risk of being associated with Reye's syndrome. However, an exception has to be made in cases of Kawasaki disease and some other symptoms. Since children of Kawasaki disease will be using aspirin for several months, it is important to take vaccination against influenza and varicella. Otherwise, these infections may cause Reye's syndrome. High dose of aspirin can cause anemia and usually dos not a deliberate advantage to disease outcomes.

When other options of treatment fail to deliver desired output or the symptoms reappear, corticosteroids is being used. The dose is usually determined in a randomized controlled trial. However, the addition of corticosteroids to aspirin and immune globulin cannot improve the outcome.

In addition, the use of corticosteroid in the setting of Kawasaki disease is correlated with the increased risk of coronary artery aneurysm. Therefore, its use in the setting is normally questioned. In the case of patients suffering from Kawasaki disease which is refractory to IVIG, it has been investigated that plasma exchange and cyclophosphamide can be possible treatment options with variable results.

Coronary lesions can be prevented in the mouse KD model by using IL-1 Receptor antagonist (anakinra). This prevention has been proved to be effective in mice even with a delay of 3 days in treatment. Nowadays, treatments do exist for iritis and other eye complications. Another option of treatment can be the inclusion of infliximab. This medicine acts by binding the tumor necrosis factor alpha.

Prognosis of KD

If treatment is done at an early stage, then there is a chance of rapid recovery from the acute symptoms, and the risk of getting coronary artery aneurysms is highly reduced. Even if the patient is not treated, the patient will eventually recover from the acute symptoms of Kawasaki disease is self-limited. However, this kind of patient is highly prone to developing coronary artery complications.

On average, about 2% of the children die from the complications involving coronary vasculitis. Patients who are diagnosed with Kawasaki disease should do an echocardiogram every few weeks at the beginning, and then continue doing it every one or two years to detect progression of any possible cardiac involvement.

Evidence has been found from the laboratory experiments about increased inflammation in combination with the demographic features, such as age greater than 8 years or less than 6 months and male gender, and also, incomplete response to IVIG therapy may result in a profile of a high-risk patient with Kawasaki disease.

The possibility that an aneurysm will resolve seems to be based on a large measure by its initial size, in which the smaller aneurysms have a greater chance of regression. Other factors are related to the regression of aneurysms in a positive way which includes fusiform rather than saccular aneurysm morphology, being younger than a year old at the start of Kawasaki disease, and a location of an aneurysm in a distal coronary segment.

Patients who develop giant aneurysms are more prone to have the highest rate of progression to stenosis. The worst case of prognosis can be seen in children suffering from large aneurysms. If this happens, then it becomes vital to do advanced treatments including coronary artery stenting, cardiac transplantation, percutaneous transluminal angioplasty, and even bypass grafting.

Soon after the initial treatment with IVIG, there is a slight chance of experiencing a relapse of symptoms. If this happens, then patients need to be hospitalized and do the treatments again. Some of the side-effects of treating with IVIG include fluid overload, aseptic meningitis, and non-allergic and allergic acute reactions. Generally, therapy for Kawasaki disease does not cause any life-threatening complications, especially compared with the risk of not treating the patient. Moreover, evidence shows that Kawasaki disease results in altered lip metabolism that stays on beyond clinical resolution of the disorder.

Epidemiology of KD

As stated earlier, Kawasaki disease affects boys more than the girls. The children who are most susceptible to the disease are of Asian ethnicity, especially of Korean, Afro-Caribbean and Japanese people. The disorder is rarely seen in Caucasians, until the last few decades. However, the rate of incidence fluctuates from one country to another.

In recent time, Kawasaki disease is the most diagnostic pediatric vasculitis found in the world. So far, the highest occurrence of Kawasaki disease is seen in Japan, with the most recent investigation placing the attack rate at 218.6 per 100,000 children in less than 5 years of age, that is, about 1 in 450 children. At this rate, presently more than 1 in 150 children in Japan are assumed to be suffering from Kawasaki disease during their lifetime.

In the United States, however, this rate of incidence is increasing day by day. Predominantly, Kawasaki disease is found in young children, having 80% of children younger than the age of 5 years. Each year in the United States, around 2000 to 4000 cases are reported and it is also evident that 9 to 19 per 100000 patients are younger than 5 years of age.

On the other hand, in the United Kingdom estimated the rate of incidence vary because of the rarity of Kawasaki disease among the children of the United Kingdom. Nonetheless, it is believed that less than 1 in every 25000 people gets affected by this disease. From the year 1991 to 2000, the rate of incidence of this disorder doubled, with 4 cases per 100000 children in 1991 compared to an increase of 8 cases per 100000 in 2000.

Pathophysiology of KD

In spite of the significant mucocutaneous clinical findings that describe the condition, Kawasaki disease is best regarded as a generalized vasculitis that includes all small to medium sized arteries. Vasculitis can also form in larger arteries, veins, small arterioles, and capillaries.

In the most primitive stages of the illness, the vascular media and the endothelial cells turn edematous, although the internal elastic lamina stays intact. Around 7 to 9 days after the beginning of the fever, an influx of neutrophils forms which is almost immediately followed by a proliferation of immunoglobulin A–producing plasma cells and CD8+ (cytotoxic) lymphocytes.

The inflammatory cells secrete different types of cytokines (vascular endothelial growth factor, tumor necrosis factor, monocyte chemotactic and activating factor), interleukins (ILs; ie, IL-1, IL-4, IL-6), and matrix metalloproteinases (MMPs; ie, primarily MMP3 and MMP9) that aim the endothelium cells and cause a cascade of events that eventually results in vascular damage and fragmentation of the internal elastic lamina.

In the vessels which are severely affected, the media results in inflammation with necrosis of smooth muscle cells. There is a chance that the external and internal laminae can split which may result in aneurysms.

During the upcoming few weeks and to months, the active inflammatory cells get replaced with monocytes and fibroblasts, and fibrous connective tissue starts to develop within the wall of the vessel. The intima becomes thick and proliferates. Eventually, the wall of the vessel becomes narrowed or blocked due to thrombus or a stenosis. Cardiovascular death may take place due to rupture of a giant coronary aneurysm or from a myocardial infarction secondary to thrombosis of a coronary aneurysm.

Many of the pathologies of the Kawasaki disease are induced by a medium vessel arterial vasculitis. At the beginning, there is an abundance of neutrophils, but the infiltrate quickly changes to plasma cells of T lymphocytes, mononuclear cells, and immunoglobulin A (IgA). All the 3 layers are involved in the inflammation. Preferentially, eosinophils are stored in microvessels.

The duration of the greatest vascular damage is when an affiliated progressive enhance in the serum platelet count takes place, and this is the moment of illness when the risk of death is the highest.

Brain natriuretic peptide (BNP), endothelin-1 (ET-1), N-terminal pro-brain natriuretic peptide and pentraxin 3 (PTX3) are generated and secreted from vascular and/or myocardial tissue. They are also very helpful in predicting the formation of coronary artery lesions and IVIG non-responsiveness and in the acute phase of the Kawasaki disease. Moreover, some biomarkers can help evaluate convalescent phase of Kawasaki disease, atherosclerosis, and chronic coronary arteritis.

Etiology of KD

The etiology of the Kawasaki disease is still unknown to people. At present, most of the immunologic and epidemiologic evidence reveals that the agent that is causing all the problems is probably infectious. Nevertheless, genetic predisposition and autoimmune reactions have been proposed to be a possible etiological factor. By the year 2016, genome-wide studies have suggested a correlation of six genetic loci to Kawasaki disease. However, the etiology of Kawasaki disease is very complex and these genetic factors still require to be completely applied to treatment and diagnosis.

In 2007, the United States Food and Drug Administration (FDA) needed the makers of RotaTeq rotavirus vaccine to make a report in the package pullout that nine cases of Kawasaki disease had been diagnosed in children who had taken the vaccine. But most of the people believed that there is no possible link between the disease and the vaccine. There was one report made about a case where an infant of 35 days old got Kawasaki disease after his second round of hepatitis B vaccination.

Infection

Some of the characteristic features of Kawasaki disease that are constant with an etiology include the formation of epidemics particularly in late winter and spring with intervals of three years and the wavelike geographic blowout of those epidemics , the self-limited characteristic of the disease and the distinctive fever, eye signs and adenopathy. Kawasaki disease is uncommon in children below 4 months of age which suggests that maternal antibodies may give passive immunity from the disorder. According to the epidemiologic data, it suggests that transmission of the disease from one person to another is not likely to happen.

Some of the authors have presented a controversial talk about the association of Kawasaki disease with recent carpet cleaning, the use of a humidifier in the room of a child with an antecedent respiratory disease, places near areas of water, and flooding. This information has led to a hypothesis of a waterborne vector.

The total clinical signs and symptoms of children with Kawasaki disease are similar to that of patients with a superantigenic or viral condition. However, studies have revealed that the immune response in Kawasaki disease is oligoclonal. This is found as a response to a usual antigen, rather than polyclonal, as would be seen in a response of a superantigen.

Multiple infectious agents have been concerned over the years. However, in recent times, no single microbial agent has been proved to be the principal cause. Infections and suspected pathogens have been enlisted in the following:

- Bacterial toxin–mediated superantigens
- MYCOPLASMA PNEUMONIAE
- Human lymphotropic virus infection
- Mite-associated bacteria
- Tick-borne diseases
- RICKETTSIA species
- PROPIONIBACTERIUM ACNES
- KLEBSIELLA PNEUMONIAE bacteremia
- Adenovirus
- Cytomegalovirus
- Parainfluenza types 3 virus
- Rotavirus infection
- Measles

- Epstein-Barr virus

- Parvovirus B19

- Meningococcal septicemia

The advantages of using light and electron microscopy have enabled the researchers to trace cytoplasmic inclusion bodies that contain RNA in 25% of adult controls and 85% of acute and late-stage Kawasaki disease fatalities. Based on this information, it is hypothetically believed that the infective agent of Kawasaki disease is most probably a pervasive RNA virus that causes asymptomatic infection in many individuals, but leads to Kawasaki disease in a subclass of genetically predisposed people.

It is hypothesized that the virus enters the body via a respiratory route, activating both the inborn and adaptive immune system. This results in B lymphocytes switching to immunoglobulin A (IgA) lymphocytes. The definition of this virus or group of other similar viruses is still under inquiry.

Genetic factors

A genetic tendency to Kawasaki disease has been suspected for a long time. Siblings of the patients have a 10 to 20 times higher chance of getting Kawasaki disease than the general people, and child patients of Japan whose parents were patients of Kawasaki disease are more likely to get more serious kind of the disease and to be more sensitive to relapse.

The risk of 2 family members with Kawasaki disease is most seen in twins, for whom the rate of suffering from the harmful effects is around 13%.

In 1978, Kato et al proved scientifically that patients with Kawasaki disease are more prone to define HLA-Bw22J2, which is a significant histocompatibility complex antigen found primarily in Japanese masses, hence, further associating a genetic influence on the enhanced sensitivity to Kawasaki disease in Japanese children. A genome-wide connection of affected brother and sister pairs was carried out in Japan, and a multipoint connection investigation found evidence of relation on chromosome 12q24.

Newburger et al, Burns et al, and Dergun et al explained families with many members affected with Kawasaki disease. In these families, Kawasaki disease attacked in 2 generations or in many siblings. No obvious sequence of inheritance could be assumed from these lineages. Therefore, multiple polymorphic alleles may influence Kawasaki disease sensitivity.

It has been found that a functional polymorphism of the inositol 1, 4, 5-triphosphate 3-kinase C (ITPKC) gene over the band 19q13.2 is very much associated with an increased sensitivity to get Kawasaki disease. Moreover, this polymorphism was linked with an increased risk of coronary artery lesions in children of both United States and Japanese ethnicity.

In a Dutch regiment, Breunig et al perceived a link between Kawasaki disease with common genetic variations in the chemokine receptor gene cluster CCR3-CCR2-CCR5. The link of CCR2-CCR5 haplotypes and CCL3L1 copy number with responses to intravenous immunoglobulin, Kawasaki disease, and coronary artery lesions have been known to be diagnostically reported in Japanese children and in other child patients too.

According to a genome research done by Taniguchi et al, the genetic factors may cause the progress of coronary artery lesions in Kawasaki disease. In the observation, genomic DNA was mined from the whole blood taken from 56 patients with Kawasaki disease who took gamma globulin treatment, and the genotypes for Fcg RIIIb-NA(1,2), Fcg RIIa-H/R131, and Fcg RIIIa-F/V158 were found.

Around 23 % of children with the HH allele for the FcgRIIa polymorphism suffered from coronary artery lesions, compared with 60% having the HR and RR alleles. HH and HR alleles may be fortune-teller of the development of coronary artery lesions in Kawasaki disease prior to the onset of gamma-globulin therapy. In addition, a polymorphism in plasma platelet-activating factor acetylhydrolase is associated with prevention to immunoglobulin treatment in Kawasaki disease.

Chapter 5- Preparation for An Appointment

Your first thought might be to make an appointment with a doctor you're familiar with or even a pediatrician but sometimes your child can be turned over to more capable hands; a pediatric cardiologist who is well experienced with employing his practice on children's hearts.

Appointments do not last forever. In a short span of time you have to convey a lot to the practician and thus, it pays to prepare beforehand. In order to help you prepare for the appointment as well as what you may expect from the doctor, here's some information.

What You Can Do?

- **Note down all the signs and symptoms your child is experiencing,** even those ones that may not seem to be related to the disease. Keep track of how frequently your child experiences fever, the temperature during that time and the duration of fever.

- **Enlist all the medications and drugs of your child,** including all minerals, vitamins, and other supplements your child is taking.

- **Take a family member or a friend to accompany you to the doctor's appointment,** if you can. It is not always possible to remember everything your doctor says. You can take a family member or a friend with you so that you don't miss out any information given during an appointment. An extra pair of ears is always better than one.

- **Note down all the questions or queries to ask your doctor.** Since your time is limited, you might want to write all your questions to save time from most important ones to least important. You may also as other questions during your talk. In case of Kawasaki disease, some basic questions to ask your child's physician or doctor include:

- What are the possible causes of the child's symptoms?

- Are there any other reasons behind the symptoms?

- Does the child require doing any test?

- How long will the child suffer from the symptoms?

- What are the available treatments, and which ones does the doctor recommend?

- What are the potential side effects of the treatments?

- Is there anything that can be done at home to make the child more comfortable?

- What are the signs and symptoms to look for in case the condition gets worst?

- What is the child's long-term prognosis of the disease?

- Do you need to follow any brochure or specific website? Furthermore, besides the enlisted ones you can also ask others questions that may come up to your mind during the appointment.

What to Expect from the Doctors?

You will probably be flooded by the doctor's questions about your child. Being prepared to answer can save time and help you devote that very time to elaborate on any points you want to go through more. The doctor may ask:

- When did symptoms start cropping up?

- How high is the fever? How long did the fever last? How severe are the symptoms?

- How to improve the symptoms?

- How will the symptoms get worse?

- Is the child being exposed to any infection or disease?

- Does the child have any kind of allergy?

What You Can Do in the Meantime?

At the beginning, your child can consume ibuprofen (Advil, Children's Motrin, others) or acetaminophen (Tylenol, others) to lessen the fever and make the child okay. However, these medicines are not advised for low temperatures, and taking these will make it difficult to determine the severity and the duration of the fever. In addition, you should never make you child take aspirin without the doctor's consultation. In teenager and young children, consuming aspirin for some viral infections, like chickenpox, can cause Reye's syndrome (a rare but dangerous disorder). The treatment for Kawasaki disease is an uncommon exception that can be made against using aspirin, but this can be under the doctor's supervision.

Conclusion

Kawasaki disease (KD) is real and its effects are devastating if left untreated. Children can't express what they're feeling most of the time. Thus, it is up to adults to keep a close watch on any new symptoms of a growing ailment. Kawasaki diseases' effects usually catch on later in life but it takes root in our childhood. If you spot symptoms like unabated high fever or conjunctivitis then take your child for a full check-up as treating Kawasaki disease within the first 2 weeks of affliction can greatly reduce the chance of any long-term harmful effects. Being a unique disease its origin has eluded us. However children that receive treatment recover fast and all we have to do then is help get them back into their lives. Soon most of the effects will dissipate and your child will just think of the experience as a bad dream.

The author would be really appreciated if you rate this book on Amazon.com! Thank you!

Made in the USA
Las Vegas, NV
09 March 2024

86946683R00030